EMBRACING

BODIES

Overcoming Body Shaming and Cultivating Body Positivity

By

Steve k. Bryant

Copyright

Contents

Chapter One

Introduction

Body shaming has become a more common problem in today's connected society, when social media platforms rule our everyday lives and pictures of perfect bodies appear on screens. People of different ages and origins encounter scrutiny and judgment because of their looks, ranging from innocuous remarks made in passing to overt complaints in public spaces. This chapter provides an overview of the intricate world of body shaming and the transformational potential of adopting a body positive mindset.

Recognizing how common body shaming is in contemporary culture

Body shaming has affected people of all demographics and penetrated many facets of society. The temptation to live up to false beauty standards can be tremendous, stemming from media representations, society norms, or interpersonal encounters. Through an examination of the frequency of body shaming, we reveal the widespread extent of this problem and its profound effects on mental health and overall wellbeing.

Social media's effect on how people perceive their bodies

Social media platforms have a big impact on how we see ourselves and other people in the digital era. These platforms' carefully chosen photos and edited lives frequently uphold limited notions of beauty, which exacerbate emotions of inferiority and comparison. By looking at how social media shapes people's opinions of their bodies, we can learn more about the processes that allow body shaming to spread and the negative impacts it has on self-esteem.

Presenting body positivity as a potential remedy

In the face of the pervasive body-shaming culture, the idea of body positivity shines as a source of empowerment and hope. Body positivity, which is based on the idea that every person deserves to be loved and respected for their body, inspires people to embrace their individuality and defy social standards. We provide readers with a foundation for a path towards self-acceptance and freedom from the constraints of unattainable beauty standards by introducing them to the ideas of body positivity.

This chapter lays the groundwork for a thorough analysis of body shaming and the transformational power of adopting a body positive approach by exploring these important issues. Through shedding light on the prevalence and effects of body shaming in contemporary culture, we enable readers to set out on a path towards self-awareness, acceptance, and empowerment.

Chapter Two

Exploring Body Shaming

In all of its manifestations, body shaming is a widespread social problem that impacts people of all ages, genders, and socioeconomic backgrounds. This chapter delves further into the idea of body shaming, breaking down its meanings, looking at its history, and analyzing the various ways it affects people's mental and emotional health.

Defining Body Shaming
At its core, body shaming involves the act of humiliating or criticizing someone based on their physical appearance. This can manifest in numerous ways, from overt comments about weight or size to subtle gestures and non-verbal cues that convey disapproval or disdain. By providing a comprehensive definition of body

shaming, we lay the groundwork for understanding its various manifestations and the harm it inflicts on individuals' self-esteem.

Examining the Forms of Body Shaming

Body shaming is not a one-size-fits-all phenomenon; rather, it manifests in diverse forms that target individuals for different aspects of their appearance. From fat shaming, which denigrates individuals for their weight or size, to skinny shaming, which criticizes thinness or lack of curves, and appearance-based shaming, which encompasses judgments about physical features beyond weight, each form of body shaming perpetuates harmful stereotypes and ideals. By examining these distinct forms, we shed light on the nuanced ways in which body shaming operates in society and its detrimental effects on individuals' self-image and confidence.

Analyzing the Causes of Body Shaming.
The roots of body shaming are deeply intertwined with societal norms, cultural expectations, and historical precedents that valorize certain body types while stigmatizing others. Media representations, celebrity culture, and beauty standards propagated by industries like fashion and entertainment play a significant role in shaping perceptions of idealized bodies, contributing to the normalization of body shaming behaviors. Additionally, personal insecurities, internalized biases, and social conditioning further fuel the cycle of body shaming, creating a toxic environment in which individuals feel pressured to conform to unrealistic standards of beauty. By analyzing the causes of body shaming, we gain insight into the underlying factors driving this harmful behavior and the systemic changes needed to address it.

Exploring the Impact of Body Shaming

The effects of body shaming extend far beyond surface-level criticisms, permeating individuals' mental and emotional well-being in profound ways. From diminished self-esteem and body dissatisfaction to the development of eating disorders and mental health issues like depression and anxiety, the consequences of body shaming can be devastating. Moreover, body shaming perpetuates a cycle of shame and self-criticism, reinforcing negative beliefs about one's worth and perpetuating harmful behaviors like disordered eating and extreme dieting. By exploring the impact of body shaming, we highlight the urgency of addressing this pervasive issue and fostering a culture of acceptance and respect for all bodies.

Through an in-depth exploration of body shaming, this chapter illuminates the complex dynamics at play in our society's attitudes towards physical appearance. By dissecting its definitions, examining its roots, and exploring its impact, we pave the way for a deeper understanding of this multifaceted issue and the transformative potential of embracing body positivity.

Chapter Three

The Three Types of Body Shaming

Body shaming is not a single, homogenous phenomenon; rather, it takes several different forms that single out victims according to particular physical characteristics. This chapter delves into the three main categories of body shaming: appearance-based shaming, slim shaming, and fat shaming. We examine how these types of shaming develop, what effect they have, and how they affect people's wellbeing and sense of self.

Fat Shaming: Probably the most well-known type of body shaming, fat shaming involves dehumanizing and stigmatizing those who are thought to be overweight or obese. This kind of body shaming frequently manifests as cruel remarks, taunting, or bullying directed at someone because of their size or weight. Fat shaming marginalizes those who do not meet these criteria while maintaining damaging stereotypes and ideas about body size. It equates thinness with worthiness and attractiveness. Furthermore, the psychological and emotional effects of fat shaming can be substantial, leaving victims with low self-esteem, feelings of humiliation, and self-hatred.

Skinny Shaming: Although it is less well-known, skinny shaming is a type of body shaming that targets those who are thought to be underweight or overly thin. Slender shaming originates from a different set of cultural expectations and ideas about beauty and attractiveness than fat shaming, which frequently results from society norms that valorize thinness. People who experience skinny shaming may be made fun of or criticized for their apparent fragility or lack of curves, which feeds negative body image stereotypes and unattainable beauty standards. Similar to fat shaming, slim shaming can be harmful to people's mental and emotional health, resulting in disordered eating patterns, feelings of inadequacy, and dissatisfaction with one's physique.

Appearance-Based Shaming: This type of shaming extends beyond comments and evaluations centered on a person's height or weight to include a wider variety of physical characteristics. Comments or criticisms on physical characteristics, such as height, hair color, facial features, or body form, are examples of this kind of shaming. The practice of appearance-based shaming upholds cultural standards and expectations regarding beauty and attractiveness, so fostering a culture of evaluation and contrast that erodes people's confidence and sense of self-worth. Appearance-based shaming, which includes disparaging someone's height, critiquing their facial characteristics, or making disparaging comments about their body type, creates a toxic atmosphere where people feel under pressure to meet rigidly prescribed ideals of beauty.

Through an examination of the three main forms of body shaming, which are appearance-based shaming, slim shaming, and fat shaming, we may better comprehend the intricate dynamics underlying societal perceptions of physical appearance. We can start challenging damaging stereotypes and ideals, fostering empathy and understanding, and promoting a culture of acceptance and respect for all bodies, regardless of size, shape, or appearance, by critically analyzing and examining various forms of shame.

Chapter four

The Impact of Body Shaming on Teens

Adolescents are especially sensitive to the negative impacts of body shaming since adolescence is a time of substantial physical, emotional, and social changes. This chapter looks at the particular difficulties that teenagers have managing peer pressure, media influences, and society expectations. It also looks at the effects that body shaming has on teens' mental health, self-esteem, and body image.

Adolescents' Susceptibility to Body Shaming

People go through major bodily changes during adolescence as they make the journey from childhood to adulthood. These alterations, in conjunction with the great pressure to meet society's ideals of beauty, have the potential to foster behaviors that involve body shaming. Teenagers may feel more self-conscious about their bodies than adults do, which makes them more vulnerable to criticism and condemnation from friends, family, and the media. Teenagers are especially susceptible to the damaging impacts of body shaming on their self-esteem and self-image since they are still developing their identities and sense of self-worth.

Social media, peers, and family influence

Teens' contacts with classmates, family, and social media have a big impact on the attitudes and views they have about their bodies and self-worth. Through their own attitudes and practices around food, exercise, and body image, parents and other caregivers have a significant influence on how teens perceive their bodies. Because teenagers frequently compare themselves to their friends and classmates and look to their social circles for approval and validation, peers can have a big impact. The emergence of social media has also brought up new difficulties, since sites like Instagram and TikTok present carefully edited pictures of idealized bodies, which can heighten emotions of inadequacy and encourage body-shaming actions.

Effects on Body Image and Self-Esteem

Teens' self-esteem and body image may suffer significant and enduring effects as a result of body shaming. Teens who experience body shaming may absorb unfavorable ideas about their bodies, which can result in emotions of guilt, worthlessness, and humiliation.

Consequently, there is a higher chance of disordered eating patterns, sadness, and anxiety when low body image and body dissatisfaction occur. Furthermore, body shaming can undermine teenagers' self-worth and confidence, making it more difficult for them to succeed academically, socially, and emotionally.

Techniques to Promote a Positive Body Image

Even though body shaming is common in society, parents, teachers, and other caregivers can help kids develop good body images by lessening the negative effects of this behavior. Promoting candid conversations about media literacy, self-worth, and body image can help youth develop resilience against temptations to shame their bodies and critically assess society's ideals of beauty. Furthermore, encouraging a culture of tolerance, acceptance, and respect for all bodies can contribute to the development of a positive atmosphere where teenagers feel appreciated and accepted for who they are rather than being made fun of for their appearance.

Through an examination of the effects of body
Shaming on teenagers' mental health, self-worth, and body image, this chapter illuminates the distinct difficulties adolescents encounter when managing social demands and media influences. We may endeavor to create a more accepting and inclusive atmosphere where teenagers feel empowered to accept their bodies and develop healthy self-esteem and body image by raising knowledge and understanding.

Chapter five

Symptoms and Effects of Body Shaming

Body shaming is a widespread problem in society that can negatively impact people's mental, emotional, and physical health. This chapter delves into the signs and consequences of body shaming, looking at how it shows up in people's attitudes, emotions, and actions as well as how it affects their general well-being and standard of living.

Understanding the Symptoms of Body Shaming

Body shaming can take many forms, both on the outside and within. Externally, people could encounter direct criticism, jeers, or harassment on their looks from other people. Internalized body shaming can take the form of self-criticism, negative self-talk, and worthlessness or inadequacy sentiments. It's critical to recognize these indicators in order to spot instances of body shaming and take appropriate action to resolve them.

Impacts on Emotional and Mental Health
Body shaming can have significant and long-lasting impacts on people's mental and emotional health. Body shaming causes people to internalize negative attitudes about their bodies and feel guilty, ashamed, and worthless, which has been related to higher levels of stress, anxiety, and depression. Furthermore, body shaming can undermine one's sense of self-worth and confidence, making it more difficult for

victims to achieve their objectives and meaningful relationships.

Effects on the Body

Body shaming can have an impact on a person's physical health in addition to their mental and emotional wellbeing. Research has indicated that long-term stress, which can be brought on by body shaming, can be linked to a number of physical health conditions, such as immunological dysfunction, digestive disorders, and cardiovascular disease. Furthermore, body shaming may make people more likely to participate in unhealthy habits like substance misuse, disordered eating, and self-harm, which could endanger their physical health and wellbeing.

The emergence of eating disorders

The link between body shaming and the emergence of eating disorders, including binge-eating disorder, bulimia nervosa, and anorexia nervosa, is among the most worrisome consequences. Body shaming can lead to disordered eating patterns when people try to fit in with unrealistic beauty standards or deal with bad sentiments about their bodies. The severe effects that eating disorders can have on a person's physical and mental health as well as their general quality of life underscore the pressing need to address body shaming as a public health concern.

Ending the Body Shaming Cycle

In order to disrupt the cycle of body shaming and lessen its negative impacts on people's health and wellbeing, activism, education, and awareness campaigns that question social norms and encourage body acceptance and self-love are crucial. This entails promoting an environment that values diversity, inclusivity, and respect for all bodies—regardless of their size, shape, or appearance—as well as offering assistance and resources to those who have been the victims of body shaming. People can regain their sense of self-worth and proudly accept their bodies if we work together to build a more compassionate and accepting society.

Chapter six

Overcoming Body Shame

Overcoming body shame is a crucial step towards self-acceptance and empowerment in the face of omnipresent societal pressures and unattainable beauty standards. This chapter looks at methods for overcoming body shame, building resilience, and promoting self-worth and a healthy body image.

Techniques to Fight Body Shame

Body shame must be overcome using a multidimensional strategy that takes into account both external and internal factors. The key to overcoming internalized body shame is to challenge negative views about one's body, practice self-compassion, and have positive self-talk. In addition, people can effectively negotiate external causes of body shame by establishing boundaries with those who engage in body shaming behaviors, surrounding themselves with affirming and supportive connections, and getting professional assistance when necessary.

Building Resilience: Resilience is the capacity to overcome hardship and face life's obstacles with grace and strength. Creating a support system, learning coping strategies, and establishing an identity and feeling of self-worth that are not dependent on approval from others are all important aspects of developing resilience in the face of body shame. People can build the resilience required to get over body shame and succeed in all facets of life by changing the way they view setbacks as opportunities for improvement, being grateful, and embracing their own talents and attributes.

Encouraging Positive Body Image and Self-Esteem: Encouraging positive body image and self-esteem entails recognizing individuality, embracing body diversity, and questioning society conventions and beauty standards. Exercise, mindfulness, and creative expression are examples of self-care activities that can assist people in reestablishing a healthy and empowering connection with their body. A more accepting and affirming society for all bodies can also be achieved by supporting organizations and programs that encourage inclusion and body acceptance, as well as by campaigning for body-positive representation in the media.

Seeking Professional Assistance: In certain situations, getting over body shame may necessitate the assistance of a licensed therapist or counselor with experience treating eating disorders and body image problems. In addition to helping people identify underlying causes of body shame, therapy can offer a secure environment in which they can explore their feelings about their bodies and create coping mechanisms for controlling unfavorable thoughts and sensations. Furthermore, online networks and support groups can provide peer support and validation to those who are having issues with their bodies, helping them feel like they belong and are not alone in their quest for self-acceptance.

Embracing Self-Love and Acceptance: The path towards self-love and acceptance is fundamental to overcome body shame. Acknowledging that genuine beauty originates from inside and accepting one's body for what it is—imperfections and all—are key components of this journey. Through self-care, healthy boundaries, and putting their health first, people can develop a strong feeling of self-acceptance and love that goes beyond what society expects of them and allows them to live truly and fully.

People can recover their feeling of self-worth and develop a healthy body image and self-esteem that enable them to flourish in all facets of life by adopting these techniques for overcoming body shame. People can overcome body shame and embrace their bodies with confidence, pride, and love by practicing self-compassion, resilience, and self-acceptance.

Chapter seven
Building Body Positivity

In an environment where unattainable beauty standards and social pressures are pervasive, promoting body positivity is a revolutionary step toward empowerment and self-love. The concepts of body positivity, techniques for cultivating a positive body image, and approaches to advancing inclusion and acceptance of all bodies are all covered in this chapter.

Recognizing the Fundamentals of Body Positivity.

Fundamentally, the ideology of body positivity is based on the idea that every body, regardless of size, shape, or appearance, is deserving of love, respect, and acceptance. The appreciation of bodily diversity and rejection of conventional beauty standards are fundamental to the body positivity philosophy. Embracing body positivity entails tearing down damaging stereotypes and expectations, questioning internalized notions of worth and beauty, and promoting an inclusive culture that values all bodies.

Self-love and self-care techniques

Building a healthy relationship with one's body and promoting body positivity require engaging in self-love and self-care practices. This means being kind and compassionate to oneself, making physical and mental health a priority, and practicing self-nourishment techniques that benefit the mind, body, and spirit. Body positivity is based on the fundamental ideas of self-love and self-care, which can be attained by mindfulness exercises, artistic expression, or self-care activities like working out and eating healthily.

Taking on Social Conventions and Beauty Standards

Body positivity places a strong emphasis on questioning society conventions and beauty standards that uphold unattainable notions of worth and attractiveness. In order to do this, one must challenge the ideas promoted by the media, advertising, and popular culture and push for more inclusive and diverse definitions of beauty. People may contribute to the creation of a more affirming and welcoming atmosphere for everyone by questioning limiting beauty standards and celebrating various bodies.

Promoting Inclusivity and Body Acceptance

Building a culture of body positivity requires promoting inclusivity and body acceptance. This entails establishing areas and societies in where every body—regardless of size, shape, or appearance—is valued and accepted. People can contribute to the creation of a more encouraging and affirming atmosphere for everyone by encouraging body acceptance and inclusivity in social settings, workplaces, and educational institutions.

Promoting Systemic Reforms
To advance body positivity on a larger scale, institutional reforms must be advocated for in addition to individual initiatives. This entails advocating for laws and programs that support inclusion and body diversity, such as inclusive fashion size standards and media representation standards that give priority to real and varied representations of beauty. Individuals can

contribute to the creation of a more inclusive and equitable society where all bodies are cherished and respected by supporting systemic improvements.

People can help create a more affirming and inclusive world where all bodies are celebrated and valued by adopting the ideas of body positivity, engaging in self-love and self-care, questioning social norms and beauty standards, encouraging body acceptance and inclusivity, and pushing for systemic changes. We can create a future where everyone feels empowered to embrace their bodies with confidence, pride, and love by promoting a culture of body positivity.

Chapter Eight

Turning Body Shaming into Body Positivity

Turning the corner towards body positivity in the face of widespread body shaming is a transforming path towards inclusivity and self-acceptance. This chapter looks at doable tactics for utilizing social media, encouraging self-expression, and pushing for structural adjustments to stop body shaming and promote a body-positive culture.

Using Social Media to Promote Change

Platforms for social media have become effective means of advancing body positivity and societal change. People can question damaging narratives, elevate underrepresented perspectives, and promote a sense of community and solidarity by utilizing body positivity hashtags, campaigns, and movements. Moreover, posting varied and genuine depictions of beauty on social media might serve as a counterbalance to the limited and exclusive representations that are promoted by the media.

Promoting Genuineness and Self-Expression

Cultivating body positivity and questioning social norms and expectations require promoting self-expression and authenticity. People can express their originality and challenge conventional definitions of beauty by embracing their distinct identity, style, and perspective. Self-expression, whether via fashion, painting, or other creative endeavors, empowers people and gives them a sense of agency, enabling them to take back control of their identities and bodies.

Promoting Systemic Reforms

While individual actions are important, tackling the underlying causes of body shaming and fostering long-lasting social change need lobbying for systemic reforms. This entails lobbying for measures that stress inclusivity and body diversity, such as body-positive education in schools, inclusive sizing in the fashion industry, and opposing discriminatory hiring and healthcare practices. Individuals can contribute to the creation of a more inclusive and equitable society where all bodies are cherished and respected by supporting systemic improvements.

Encouraging Intersectional Positive Body Image

Intersectionality acknowledges that racial, gendered, sexual, ability, and socioeconomic position are only a few of the intersecting identities that influence how people experience body shaming. Advocating for inclusive places and resources that uplift and empower all bodies, addressing the particular kinds of discrimination and oppression faced by marginalized populations, and highlighting their voices and experiences are all part of promoting intersectional body positivity. In the struggle against body shaming, people can forge a more egalitarian and inclusive movement for body positivity by emphasizing intersectionality.

Promoting Understanding and Empathy
Building unity and taking action as a group in the battle against body shaming requires cultivating empathy and understanding. People can develop empathy and compassion for those who have been oppressed or mistreated by

listening to others and validating their stories. Furthermore, learning about the social, cultural, and historical elements that contribute to body shaming can make people more adept supporters in the fight for body acceptance and help them comprehend the complexity of this problem.

People can end body shaming and create a more inclusive and affirming body positivity culture by using social media to promote positive change, encouraging self-expression and authenticity, fighting for systemic changes, supporting intersectional body positivity, and cultivating empathy and understanding. Together, we can dismantle harmful standards and advance body acceptance and respect, paving the way for a day when everyone is empowered to love, accept, and feel proud of their bodies.

Chapter Nine

Case Studies and Success Stories

This chapter explores motivational case studies and success stories of people who have accepted body positivity and triumphed over body shaming. These true stories act as rays of light and inspiration, showing how resilient living, self-acceptance, and community support can be even in the face of discrimination and social pressure.

Case Study 1: Self-Love Journey of Sarah

Sarah, a young lady who battled low self-esteem and problems with her body image, describes her path to self-acceptance and love. With the help of counseling, family support, and engagement in online body-positive networks, Sarah gained the ability to confront her negative body image and accept her own beauty and deservingness. These days, Sarah advocates for self-compassion and body acceptance, acting as a role model for those who are dealing with body shame.

Practical Tips from Sarah's Journey
Engage in self-compassion: Be nice and patient with yourself, especially when you're feeling insecure or self-conscious.

Disprove unfavorable beliefs: Determine and combat the unfavorable ideas and cognitive processes that fuel body shame.

Put self-care first: Take part in activities that feed your mind, body, and spirit, such as yoga, meditation, or artistic endeavors.

Seek assistance: Speak with dependable family members, friends, or experts who can provide direction, affirmation, and assistance on your path to self-acceptance and love.

Case Study 2: John's Experience with Fatphobia

A plus-sized man named John talks about how he has dealt with prejudice and fatphobia in a number of spheres of his life, such as dating, work, and healthcare. John was met with discrimination and stigma from society, but he chose not to let those feelings consume him. Instead, he became a vocal supporter of body positivity and fat acceptance. John strives to combat fatphobia and advance inclusivity and respect for all bodies via activism and community organization.

Practical Tips from John's Experience:
Subvert social norms: The cultural conventions and beauty standards that support discrimination and fatphobia should be questioned and challenged.

Promote change: Advocate for structural changes that support body diversity and inclusivity in all spheres of society by using your voice and platform.

Embrace a supportive environment: Be in the company of encouraging friends, family, and communities that value and appreciate various body types.

Develop self-acceptance: Accept the way your body looks and acknowledge your own beauty and worthiness despite external norms.

Case Study 3: Maya's Journey to Recovery
Maya, an eating disorder survivor, talks about her path to healing and self-awareness. Following years of battle with disordered eating patterns and a poor perception of her body, Maya sought help and started on a road to recovery and self-acceptance. Maya gained knowledge on how to value her mental and emotional health and develop a healthy relationship with her body through counseling, support groups, and self-care routines. As an advocate for body positivity and eating disorder awareness today, Maya draws on her personal experience to encourage others as they pursue recovery.

Success Story 1: The Body Positive Movement
The Body Positive Movement is a grassroots movement that aims to challenge societal beauty

standards and promote body acceptance and inclusivity for all. Through workshops, educational programs, and community outreach initiatives, The Body Positive Movement empowers individuals to embrace their bodies with confidence and pride, regardless of size, shape, or appearance. With chapters around the world, The Body Positive Movement continues to inspire and uplift individuals on their journey to self-love and acceptance.

Success Story 2: Body-Positive Brands Leading Change

A number of companies have taken the lead in the battle against body shaming by emphasizing diversity and inclusivity in their advertising campaigns and product lines. By celebrating bodies of all shapes, sizes, and identities, these brands subvert conventional notions of beauty and advance a more affirming and inclusive definition of beauty. These firms are encouraging people to accept their bodies with confidence and pride by empowering people to redefine society's ideas of beauty through the use of varied models and a diversity of body types in their advertising.

Success Story 3: Online Communities Fostering Support and Connection

People dealing with body image issues can find a lot of support and validation from online forums that promote body positivity and self-love. People can find support and encouragement on their path to self-acceptance by connecting with people who have gone through similar experiences through social media platforms, forums, and online support groups. They can also exchange resources and insights with these others. These virtual communities offer a secure environment where people can be themselves, question damaging conventions, and develop a feeling of empowerment and belonging.

We learn about the varied experiences of people who have rejected body shaming and embraced body positivity through these case studies and success stories. These narratives, which range from individual self-discovery journeys to group initiatives to question social norms, serve as a constant reminder of the resiliency, strength, and beauty that are innate to every body. By telling these stories, we give others hope and give them the confidence, pride, and love they deserve to appreciate their bodies.

Practical Tips from Maya's Journey

Seek out expert assistance: For assistance and direction, get in touch with a therapist or counselor who specializes in eating disorders and body image difficulties.

Make connections with others: Look for online forums or support groups where you may interact with people who have gone through similar things and receive encouragement and support.

Engage in self-compassion: Treat yourself with care and gentleness, especially when you're going through difficult times or facing disappointments.

Pay attention to your advantages:

Acknowledge and cherish your distinct advantages, attributes, and skills independent of your looks or stature.

To sum up, this chapter's case studies and success stories provide insightful information, important takeaways, and useful advice for eschewing body shaming and embracing body positivity. People can regain their feeling of self-worth and develop a positive relationship with their bodies by being resilient, self-compassionate, and receiving support from their communities. This will pave the way for a day when all bodies will be appreciated and celebrated.

Case Study 2: John's Experience with Fatphobia

John's battle with fatphobia serves as a reminder of the widespread prejudice and stigma that people with larger bodies must endure. Because of his stature, John experienced bullying, taunting, and marginalization from an early age, which left him feeling ashamed and self-hatred. John had obstacles throughout his life, but he chose not to let society's negative messages about his appearance affect him. Instead, he became a vocal supporter of body positivity and fat acceptance.

John has devoted countless hours to combating fatphobia and advancing inclusivity and respect for all bodies via activism and community organizing. He has advocated for structural changes that put body diversity and inclusivity first, speaking out against discriminatory policies in healthcare, employment, and media representation. By doing this, John has encouraged people to accept their bodies, no matter what size or form, with pride and confidence.

Chapter Ten
Nurturing Body Positivity in Future Generations

It is crucial to cultivate body positivity in the next generation as we work to build a society that is more accepting and supportive. In this chapter, we examine how parents, teachers, legislators, and the media can support a body-positive society and provide young people the tools they need to accept their bodies with resilience, confidence, and self-love.

Parental Guidance and Assistance: Instilling a favorable body image in their children and influencing their views toward their bodies are major responsibilities of parents. Early modeling of body positivity, self-acceptance, and self-care routines can help parents' foster resilience and self-worth in their children. Furthermore, encouraging candid conversations about media literacy, self-esteem, and body image can help give kids the skills they need to resist social pressure and develop a healthy relationship with their bodies.

Initiatives for Education and Curriculum Integration: It is crucial to incorporate body positivity education into school curriculum in order to give young people the knowledge and abilities they need to oppose damaging beauty standards and encourage body acceptance. Teachers can enable children to critically evaluate media messages, appreciate diversity, and develop resilience in the face of social pressures by introducing courses on media literacy, diversity, and self-esteem into health and wellness programs. Furthermore, encouraging inclusive and body-positive learning settings in schools can contribute to the development of a safe and encouraging environment where all children can succeed.

Advocacy and Policy Interventions: Through campaigning and legislative action, policymakers are instrumental in influencing cultural norms and advancing body positivity. A more fair and inclusive society where all bodies are appreciated and respected can be achieved by legislators by enacting laws that support body diversity and inclusivity, such as prohibiting weight-based discrimination in work and healthcare settings. Furthermore, supporting media representation policies that give priority to real and varied depictions of beauty can support the wider promotion of body acceptance and the opposition of damaging beauty standards.

Industry Accountability and Media Representation: Prioritizing inclusive and diverse representation is crucial for media makers and industry stakeholders since the media and entertainment sector have a big impact on how society views beauty and body image. Media artists may support diversity and body acceptance by showcasing a variety of identities, sizes, and body types in advertising, television, film, and other media platforms. This helps to challenge limiting ideals of beauty. Additionally, systemic change and the advancement of an inclusive and affirming media landscape can be facilitated by holding media outlets and marketers responsible for the propagation of damaging stereotypes and values.

Participation in the Community and Grassroots Activism: Local social change and the promotion of a body-positive culture depend on community involvement and grassroots effort. Grassroots activists may mobilize communities, raise awareness, and fight damaging beauty stereotypes by planning seminars, events, and campaigns centered around body acceptance and self-love. Creating helpful environments and tools, such online forums and support groups, can also help people who are having problems with their body image by offering much-needed encouragement and camaraderie on the path to self-acceptance.

We can create a more inclusive and affirming society where all bodies are celebrated and valued by fostering body positivity in future generations through parental influence and support, educational initiatives and curriculum integration, policy interventions and advocacy efforts, media representation and industry accountability, community engagement and grassroots activism. Body positivity will become the standard rather than the exception in the future when we enable youth to embrace their bodies with resilience, confidence, and self-love.

Chapter eleven

Conclusion

In this last chapter, we consider how readers might resist social conventions and embrace their individuality by reflecting on the path from body shame to body positivity. We stress the significance of working together to build a more welcoming and inclusive society where all bodies are respected and honored.

Contemplating the Trip: There will be times of hardship, self-discovery, and empowerment along the highly personal and transforming path from body shame to body positivity. People learn to accept their bodies with confidence, resiliency, and self-love as they navigate cultural constraints, internalized beliefs, and outside criticism. People reclaim their sense of self-worth and develop a positive relationship with their bodies by being resilient, self-compassionate, and receiving support from their communities. They realize that they are worthy and beautiful beyond society norms.

Giving Readers the Tools to Question Social Norms: We give readers the tools they need to question cultural norms and beauty standards that uphold discrimination and body shame while they consider their personal journeys towards body positivity. We urge readers to oppose damaging stereotypes, challenge limited conceptions of beauty, and promote diversity and representation in all spheres of society. Readers may create a more welcoming and inclusive society where all bodies are appreciated by embracing their individuality and enjoying variety.

The Value of Group Initiatives: We stress the significance of group action in bringing about systemic change and advancing body positivity on a larger scale, even though individual efforts are vital. Through uniting as a community, promoting legislative modifications, and opposing prejudicial behaviors, we may establish a fairer and more comprehensive society that values and honors every body. We can resist oppressive structures, amplify underrepresented voices, and build a future where everyone feels empowered to embrace their bodies with confidence, pride, and love by standing together, showing empathy, and becoming allies.

In summary, the transition from body shame to body positive is evidence of the strength of fortitude, compassion, and support from others in the community. All bodies are cherished and respected in a more inclusive and welcoming world that we can create by thinking back on our own experiences, questioning social standards, and pushing for change. We can create a world free from the restrictions of body shame and prejudice, where everyone feels empowered to embrace their unique self and live truthfully. We can do this by working together and showing solidarity.